Training Your Inner Pup to Eat Well

Let Your Stomach Be Your Guide

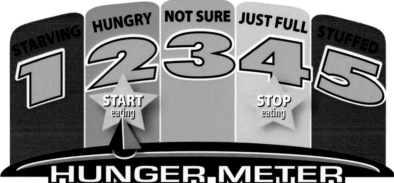

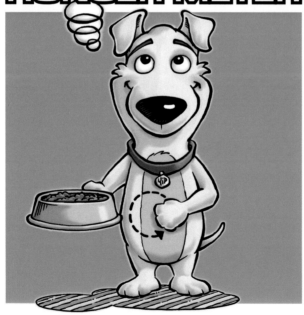

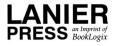

LANIER
PRESS *an Imprint of*
BookLogix

Alpharetta, GA

ISBN: 978-1-63183-203-1

Library of Congress Control Number: 2017959830

10 9 8 7 6 5 4 3 2   1 1 0 9 1 7

Printed in the United States of America

♾ This paper meets the requirements of ANSI/NISO Z39.48-1992 (Permanence of Paper)

Illustrations by Robbie Short (www.robbieshort.com)

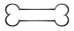

Contents

Preface

Where did Yip come from? I had been a therapist for many years, a specialist helping adults use their appetite cues to manage urges to eat, when our family adopted a young terrier named Lucy. I had never owned a dog, and I quickly found out that keeping Lucy healthy was quite different from talking to adults about their eating. Once, I left three steaks on a kitchen counter and returned a few minutes later to find a very stuffed (and ultimately sick) dog. Lucy taught me to respect the very basic nature of desire for food, becoming my inspiration for Yip.

Two of my innovative young colleagues, Dr. Nancy Zucker and Dr. Thrudur Gunnarsdóttir, started applying my work on appetite retraining to adolescents and children, encouraging me to develop the idea further. A wonderful ten-year-old boy, Tiger Greene, and his family were referred to me, and I was challenged to find more fun and effective ways to help families start their journey to better health (see his story in *Sacking Obesity*, Harper Collins, 2012). Yip became an instant hit with both the children and their parents. The idea of an adorable pup who just likes to eat is appealing and helps everyone accept the reality that it isn't really natural to limit what we eat, but it is possible to eat well and be happy. Most dog owners (including children) find they are quite able to keep their dog happy with mostly healthy food. But, many of us have a much harder time feeding ourselves (or our children) well.

I hope to carry on Tiger's efforts to help children, adolescents, and adults find a different way to think about all the choices they have to make living in a world of too many fun and tasty (but very high calorie) treats. Please give training your Yip a try; I think you will be glad you did.

Acknowledgments

I want to express my appreciation to Rex and Duval Fuqua and Fuqua family foundations for their support during the early phases of the development of this book; to my students who contributed to the development of appetite retraining over the years, my former postdocs Sheethal Reddy and Jessica Nasser, and especially Lauren Marx, Joya Hampton, Elise Obdarski, and Devika Basu, who helped shape Yip into the dog that he is today; and to my colleagues in the Department of Pediatrics, National University Hospital of Iceland, especially Sigrún Þorsteinsdóttir and Berglind Brynjólfsdóttir, who incorporated the dog concept within their Children's Obesity Clinic program and provided such valuable feedback. I also want to thank Wayne South Smith for helping me find Yip's voice, and my friend Ann Carroll for putting the finishing touches on this manuscript.

Notes for Parents

What Is Your Role?

Your child will *always* have opportunities to choose less healthy foods and to overeat, so your child must learn to manage his or her own desires to eat—a process this book calls "training *Your Inner Pup*." In the long run, your child will not be able to rely on you to limit what he or she eats. Therefore, your job is to *train the trainer*. In other words, you will be training your child to train himself. Your attitude as you do this job makes a big difference. If you can remain positive and focus on his successes, your child can learn healthier eating habits without making eating a source of tension and conflict within the family.

Your role will change depending upon the age of your child. This book is written in such a way that it can be used with a wide age range. With a young child, read the book to her often and start using some of the words when you talk about eating (do not talk about weight!). With an older child, you might ask her to read the book first and then explain to you what she thinks the book says. This puts her in the role of teacher. With a teen or young adult, just give him the book, saying you think it is an interesting way to think about why it is so hard for anyone to limit eating tasty food that is not so healthy (i.e., junk food). Let him know that you are willing to help him if he would like help. If he wants help, ask specifically what you can do that would be helpful, and also what you may be doing now that is *not* helpful. Sympathize with your child that it is a tough job to train *any* puppy, but you have confidence she will be able to train her own *Inner Pup*. Help your child make this training fun, as if your child were, in fact, responsible for caring for and training an adorable puppy with a mind of its own. You can help your child learn how to manage his or her puppy!

Remind your child often that puppies can be very different. They have different food preferences, impulses, and ways of learning. Your child may need to try many different strategies to figure out what works for her and what does *not* work. What works for one child may not work for her sibling

vi

or friend. What works may change as your child gets older or has to deal with new situations. You may need to be flexible in adapting family expectations, especially if there are other children or a parent who does not have much difficulty with weight or eating healthy. Those individuals often have a hard time understanding why a child is having difficulties with food, and they may not understand how much support the child needs to be successful in eating well. Respect your child's feelings and preferences for how to manage his *Inner Pup*, but don't let your child give you a lot of excuses for why he can't learn to manage his eating. Allow your child to take as much of the responsibility for their food choices as he can handle. Try not to let your child make his eating primarily *your* problem. The effort will wear you out, and it is less likely to be successful in the long run.

Yes, you are responsible for doing all you can to keep your child healthy, but when it comes to weight, this means helping your child take ownership of her own health—at whatever level she can manage. When you try too hard to impose your own values about being healthy and insist on your solutions to *make* her eat healthy, you risk eliciting feelings in her of being overcontrolled, feelings that are likely to sabotage your best efforts. Think about how you feel when other people try to tell you what to do instead of helping you figure out what you actually are willing to do differently. Most of us don't like being told what to do. We either tune the person out or do what we want behind their back.

As a parent, your job is to be both coach and cheerleader, to be patient and to remain positive as your child figures out how to best manage his or her own desires to eat in a world full of tempting, tasty foods.

For updates and additional information, please see
http://craigheadlab.weebly.com/.

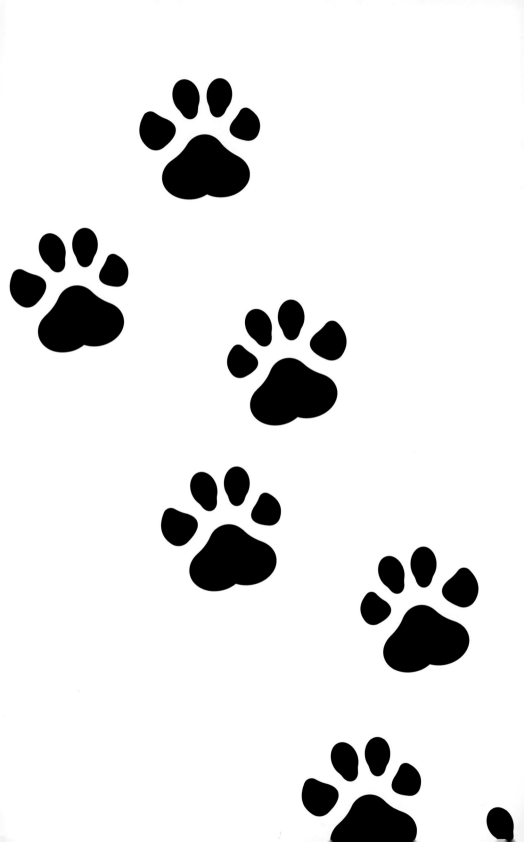

Chapter 1
Meet Yip, Your Inner Pup

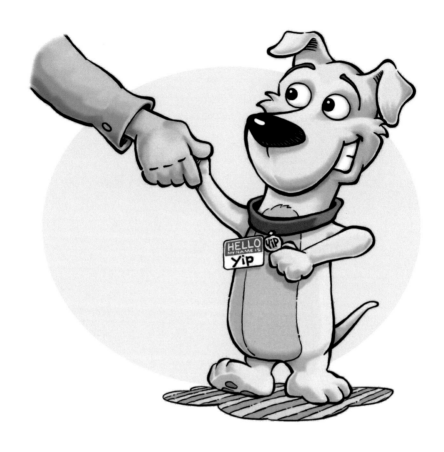

Your Inner Pup is the part of you that wants to eat. Let's call this part of you "Yip."

Puppies are hunters. Hunters eat *whenever* they find tasty food. Also, puppies don't stop and think, *Am I hungry?* Puppies don't stop and think, *Is this food nutritious?* So, puppies don't stop and think, *Am I full?*

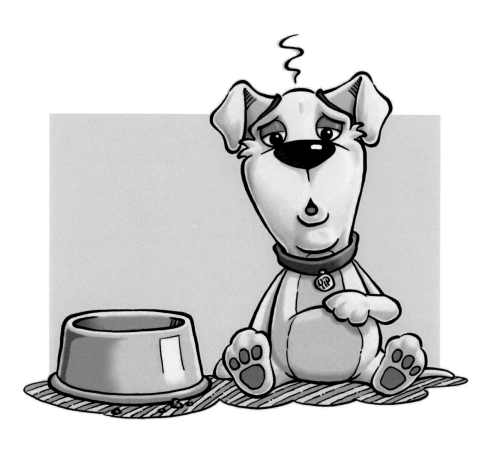

Puppies eat *as much* as they want.

Sometimes a puppy eats so much, he doesn't feel very good.

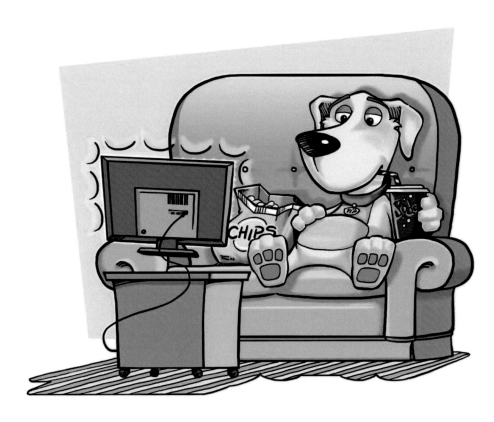

Puppies don't stay healthy if they get to eat *whatever* they want to eat or as *much* as they want.

Puppies need a trainer to keep them healthy. Yip, *Your Inner Pup,* needs a trainer too. *The Thinking You is* the part of you that is reading this book. *The Thinking You* can train Yip. Are you willing to start training Yip to eat well?

1. If you don't own a dog yourself, talk to people you know who do have a dog. Find out what they feed their dog. What foods do they feed their dog? What foods are they careful NOT to give their dog? Why don't they give their dog those foods?

2. Will their dog eat whenever they offer their dog food? Or, is their dog picky and only eats certain foods? Do they let their dog have food whenever he begs? Why don't they let their dog eat whenever he wants to, and as much as he wants to?

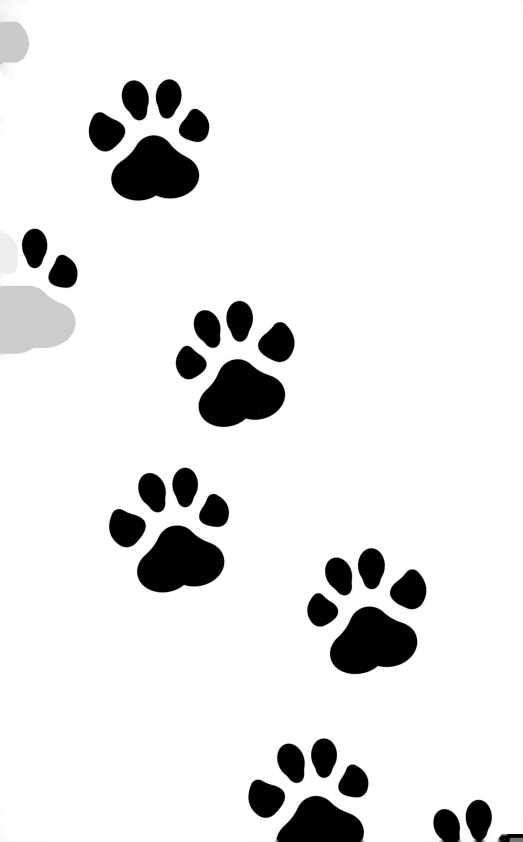

Chapter 2
How Do You Train a Puppy
to Do What's Best?

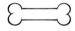

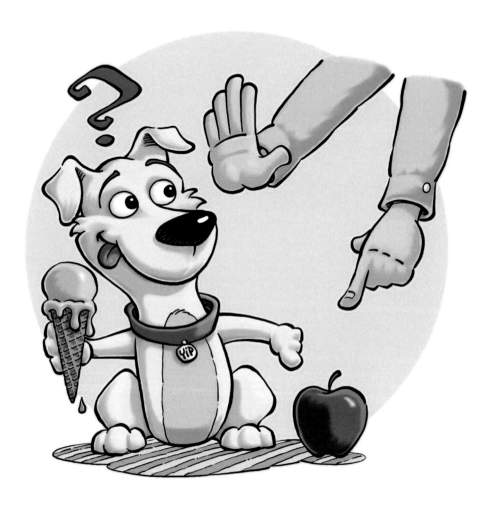

Puppies have to learn to do what their trainer wants them to do.

A trainer teaches a puppy to eat well because he loves his puppy. He wants his puppy to feel good and stay healthy for a long time. So, a trainer gives his puppy nutritious food that tastes good.

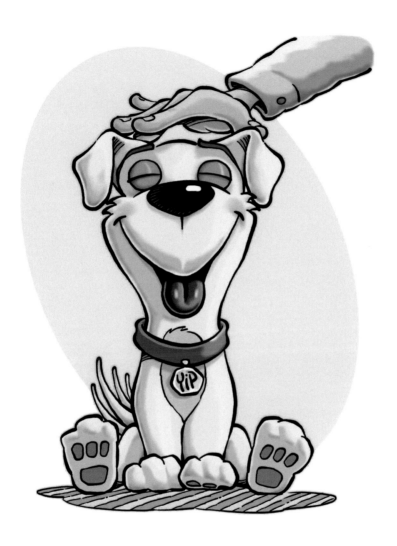

A trainer tells his puppy, "Good job!" *every time* the puppy does what the trainer thinks is best.

It is a lot of work to train a puppy, but puppies can learn to do what their trainer thinks is best. Puppies like to make their trainers happy. Puppies can learn to be happy eating well.

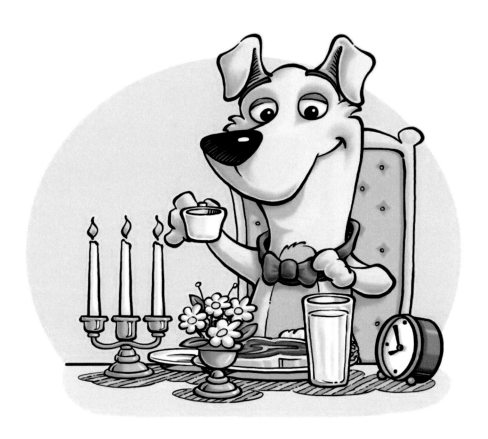

A trainer feeds his puppy nutritious meals about the same time every day.

A puppy needs regular meals so he will not get *too* hungry before it is time to eat. *Your Inner Pup* needs breakfast, a morning snack, lunch, an afternoon snack, and dinner. A puppy doesn't need a lot of treats to be happy. A puppy needs a trainer who loves him and keeps him healthy.

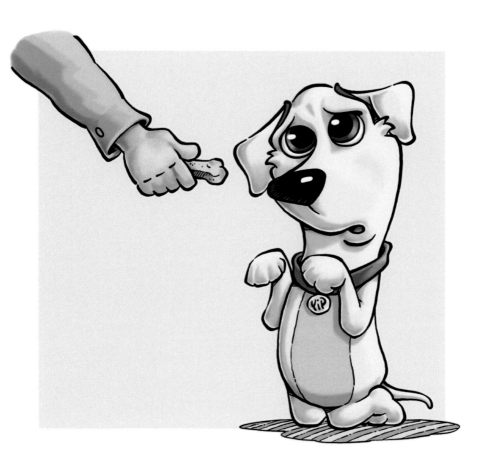

A trainer doesn't give his puppy a treat every time the puppy begs.

Treats taste really good in your mouth, and treats are a lot of fun to eat, but treats are not as good for your body as more nutritious snacks. Some treats have a lot of sugar, like a candy bar. Some treats are fried or have a lot of salt, like potato chips, french fries, and fried chicken. Trainers do give puppies small treats sometimes, just for fun. But trainers know when it is NOT the right time to give a puppy a treat.

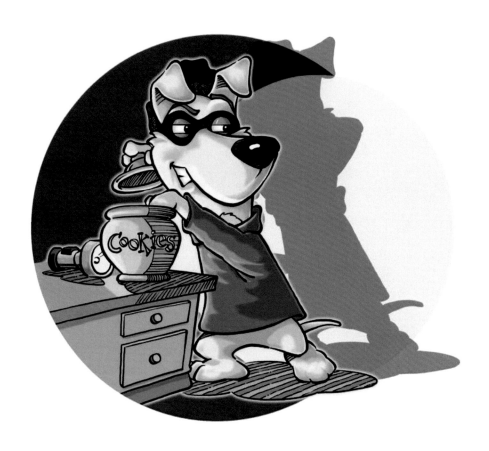

A trainer stays in charge of feeding his puppy. Puppies will sneak treats if they can.

A trainer doesn't leave treats where a puppy can find them. A trainer helps his puppy wait for the right time to get a treat. A trainer tells other people, "Don't give my puppy treats. I want to keep my puppy healthy."

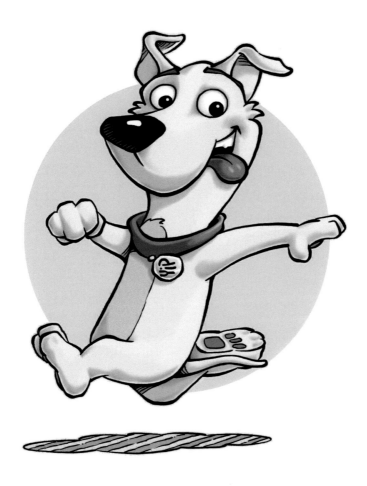

A trainer takes his puppy out to run and play.

Puppies don't need a lot of treats to be happy. Puppies do need a lot of exercise to be happy and to stay healthy. Puppies are happiest when you pet them and play with them A LOT.

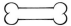

1. Have you tried to train a dog to obey commands or do tricks? How did you teach your dog to do what you wanted it to do (or not do, like jumping up on people)? Was it easy, or did it take a lot of practice? If you don't own a dog, ask people who have dogs how they train them.

2. Why does a dog learn to do what their owner wants them to do most of the time? What is important to a dog besides getting food?

Chapter 3
The Thinking You Can Train Yip
to Eat Well

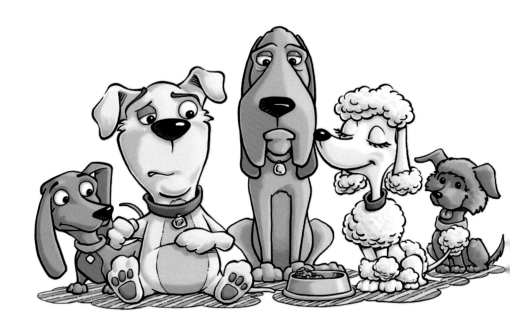

Some puppies need more practice than others.

At first, Yip won't always do what the *Thinking You* knows is best. You may get frustrated and want to stop training. It takes a lot of practice for Yip to learn healthy eating habits. Tell Yip "Good job!" when he listens to the *Thinking You*. Be patient. Once Yip learns new habits, he will feel happier making healthy choices.

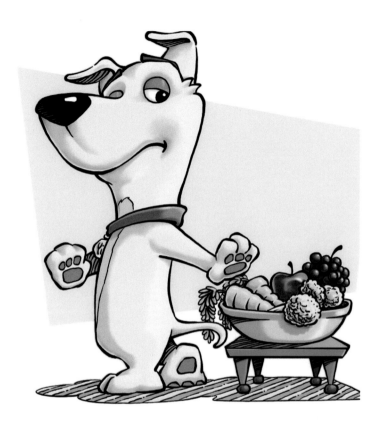

When you start training Yip, remember these tips:

The Thinking You decides WHAT KINDS of foods to give Yip.

Don't let Yip be stubborn and refuse to try different vegetables and fruits.

Ask a grown-up to help you find nutritious foods that Yip likes. Sometimes it takes a while for a puppy to get used to new foods. Tell Yip "Good job!" when he is willing to try new, nutritious foods.

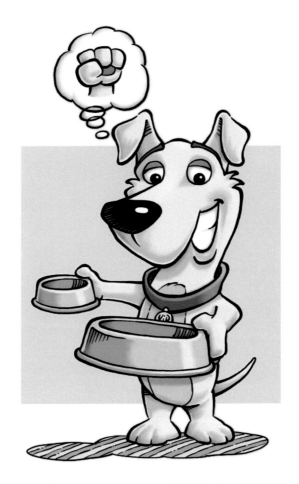

The Thinking You decides **HOW MUCH** food to give Yip.

Don't give Yip a large bowl of food. Yip's stomach is just a little larger than his fist.

Yip needs just enough food to fill his stomach, but Yip will eat as much as you give him. Yip doesn't need as much food as he *wants*. Tell Yip "Good job!" when he finds something else to do instead of asking for more food than you think is best.

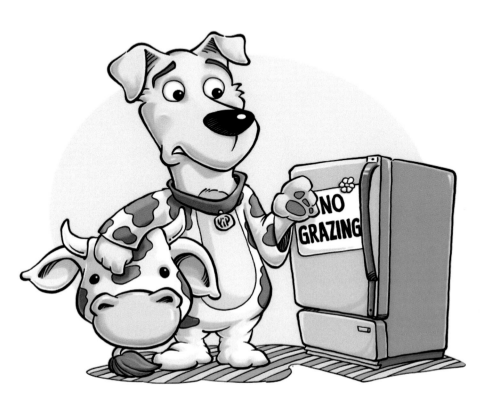

The Thinking You decides **WHEN** Yip gets snacks and treats.

Cows have to eat all day long to eat enough grass to stay healthy. Yip is not a cow.

Yip can have a nutritious snack between meals, but if Yip eats snacks all afternoon, he won't be hungry for his nutritious dinner. If Yip eats too many snacks and treats, he won't stay healthy. Tell Yip "Good job!" when he waits to eat at the right time.

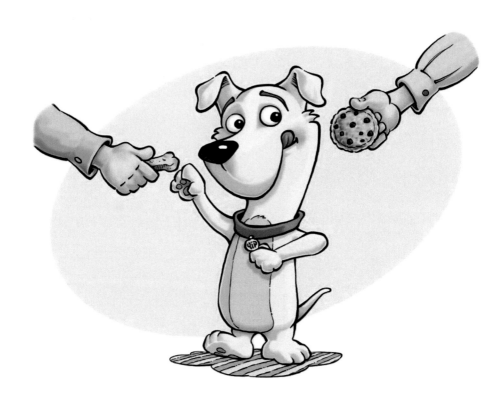

The Thinking You decides **WHO** gets to give Yip treats.

Help Yip learn when it is the right time to have a treat. Other people may offer Yip too many treats.

When Yip is not hungry, teach him to say, "NO, thank you. I don't need a treat right now. I may have a treat later." If Yip has already had enough treats, teach him to say, "I've had enough treats today. I can have another treat tomorrow if I decide I want one." Tell Yip "Good job!" when he decides he doesn't need a treat every time someone offers him one.

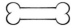

1. Write down a list of nutritious snacks that you like, and some you don't like as much but would be willing to eat more often.

2. Write down a list of foods you like to have for special treats. How much do you usually eat of these treats? Is it hard for you to eat just a small amount of some of these foods? How can you make it easier to eat only small amounts of special-treat foods? Sometimes choosing to eat individually packaged food helps, like a small bag of chips or crackers. Sometimes it helps to eat these treats when you are out of the house instead of keeping a lot of treats in your house.

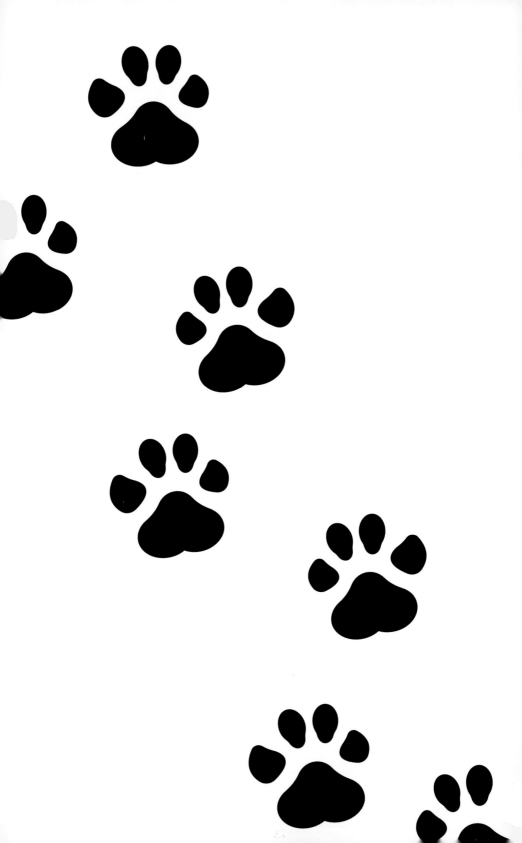

Chapter 4
Train Yip to Use the Hunger Meter

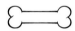

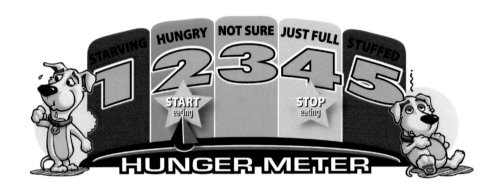

The Hunger Meter tells Yip when it is the right time to start eating, and when it is the right time to stop eating.

The *Hunger Meter* says, "Stay out of the red zones. Don't get starving and don't get stuffed."

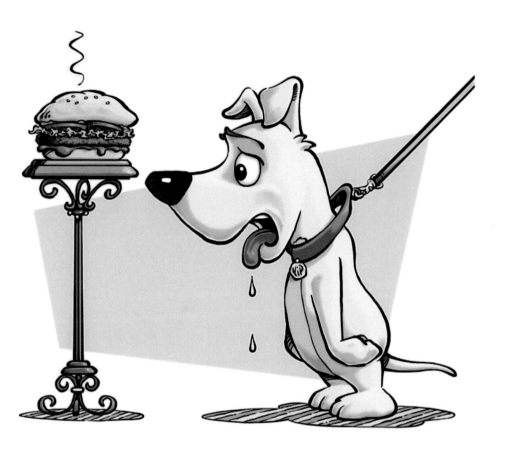

The Hunger Meter reminds Yip, "Don't skip meals or get too hungry."

When Yip is STARVING, it is hard for him to make healthy choices. A hungry puppy will eat whatever he can find. He will eat too fast and eat more than his body needs to stay healthy. When Yip is hungry, it is the *right time* to choose a nutritious meal or snack. It is NOT the *right time* to choose a treat. If Yip is *very hungry*, he will eat too much treat food. Yip can enjoy having a small treat *after* he has had a nutritious meal.

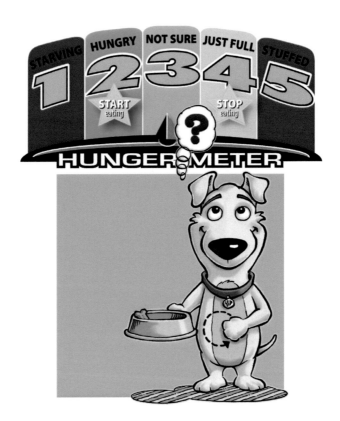

The Hunger Meter helps Yip figure out what to do when he is NOT SURE if he is hungry.

Train Yip to listen to his stomach and let his stomach be his guide. When Yip's stomach is HUNGRY, it is the *right time* to start eating. When Yip's stomach is *not* HUNGRY, it is NOT the *right time* to eat. Help Yip learn the difference between feeling hungry in his stomach and *wanting* something tasty in his mouth. When Yip is NOT SURE if he is hungry in his stomach, it is best if he finds something else fun to do and waits for his next meal or snack time.

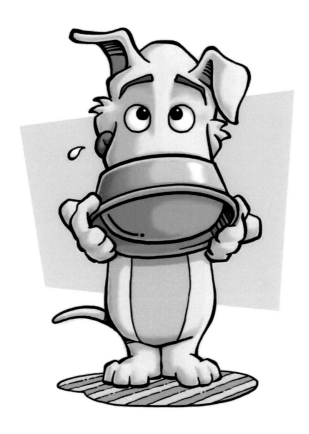

It is not a good idea for Yip to get STUFFED, even when he is eating nutritious food.

Yip needs to eat his nutritious meals, especially his vegetables, but it is not a good idea for Yip to get STUFFED, no matter what he is eating. When Yip is used to getting STUFFED with nutritious foods, he will want to get STUFFED when he is eating treats too. Help Yip listen to his stomach and find something else fun to do as soon as he is JUST FULL instead of eating as much as he can.

1. Can you "listen" to your stomach? Can you tell the difference between feeling hungry in your stomach and when you just want to eat because food tastes good in your mouth?

2. Think about a time when you had to wait a long time before you could eat. Did you eat a lot really fast when you finally got to eat? Sometimes it helps to bring your own snack if you may not have a chance to eat or if you won't be able to get a nutritious snack.

Chapter 5
Train Yip to Use
the Worth-It Scale

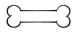

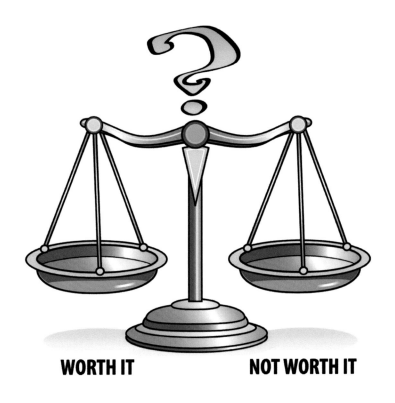

WORTH IT   **NOT WORTH IT**

Yip has to make a lot of choices about WHEN to eat, HOW MUCH to eat, and WHAT KINDS of foods to eat.

Train Yip to use the *Worth-It Scale* to compare choices. Encourage Yip to let his stomach be his guide. Some foods may taste good in his mouth, but may not feel as good in his body later on. If Yip eats a lot of sugar, he may feel very excited for a while, but he may get tired quickly. If he eats a lot of fried food, his stomach may not feel so good later. Help Yip make choices so he is happy, and he still feels good in his body after he eats.

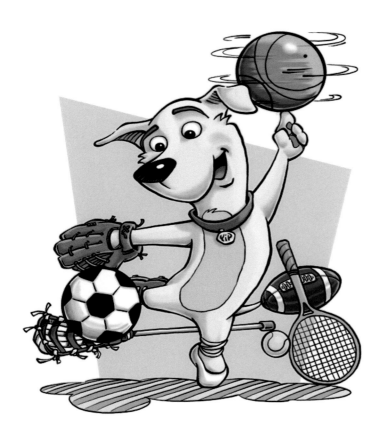

Yip's choice: Eat whenever he wants to eat, or choose something else fun to do?

Sometimes Yip just *wants* to eat. He may feel bored. He may not want to do his homework. He may want a special treat. Train Yip to stop and think: Is *this the right time to eat?* Or, *will I feel better if I find something else fun to do?*

When Yip is NOT SURE if he is hungry in his stomach, help Yip wait for his next meal or snack time. Tell Yip "Good job!" *every* time he chooses fun activities instead of eating when he is *not* HUNGRY.

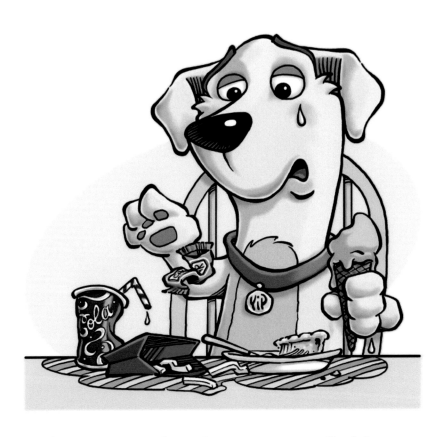

Yip's choice: Eat when he wants to feel better, or choose to do something else to feel better?

When Yip is not feeling happy, sometimes he really *wants* treats. Eating treats makes Yip feel better for a while. But, Yip may eat too many treats, and he may even feel sick later.

When Yip feels sad or upset, help him find other ways to feel better. Yip can take a walk, talk to a friend, read a book, do crafts or hobbies, dance, or play sports. Tell Yip "Good job!" *every* time he figures out another way to feel better instead of eating treats.

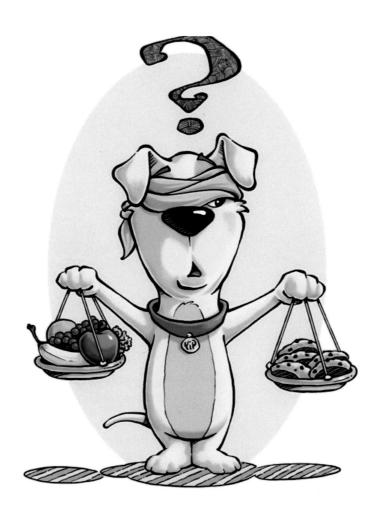

Yip's choice: Eat a *nutritious* snack, or eat treats?

Help Yip choose tasty, nutritious snacks instead of treats when his stomach feels HUNGRY. Sometimes a treat is Worth It. Treats are a fun part of life, but Yip doesn't need a treat every time he wants one. Tell Yip "Good job!" every time he chooses a nutritious snack instead of a treat.

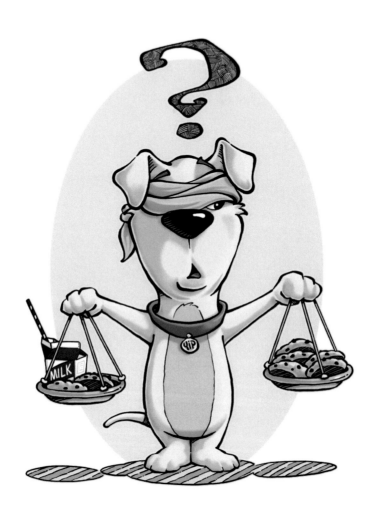

Yip's choice: Eat a small treat, or eat lots of treats?

When Yip decides it is the *right time* for a treat, help him make a healthy choice. Yip may choose two cookies with a glass of nutritious milk instead of a lot of cookies. Tell Yip "Good job!" *every* time he chooses a *small treat* instead of *a large amount of treats*.

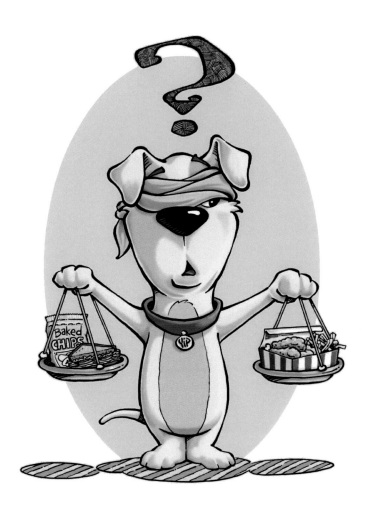

Yip's choice: Eat fried chicken with fries, or eat foods that are NOT fried?

Fried chicken and fries taste good, and Yip can eat a *small* amount sometimes, but encourage Yip to try baked chips and a sandwich more often. Tell Yip "Good job!" *every* time he chooses foods that are NOT fried instead of fried foods.

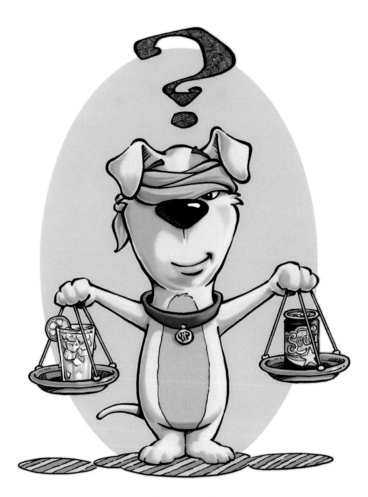

Yip's choice: Drink soda, or drink water?

Drinks with sugar taste good, but all that extra sugar is NOT healthy for your body. Even sugary juice isn't healthy. Encourage Yip to choose milk or drink water. He can add lemon slices or have flavored water. Tell Yip "Good job!" *every* time he chooses something healthy to drink instead of drinks with sugar.

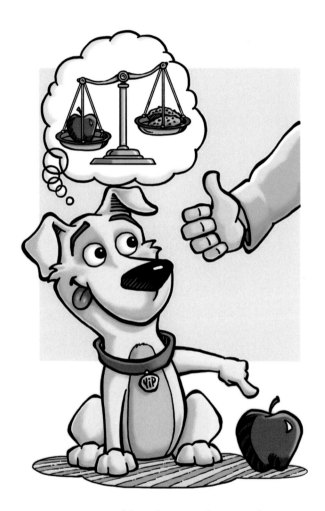

Yip is just a puppy, and he has a lot to learn. Be patient.

Yip wants the *Thinking You* to be happy, but Yip also likes treats. At first, Yip won't always do what the *Thinking You* knows is best. Keep training Yip to stop and think: *Is this choice Worth It*, or *Not Worth It*?

Yip has to practice A LOT to learn new, healthy eating habits. Tell Yip "Good job!" *every* time he makes the healthier choice. Praise makes Yip feel good and helps him want to do what the *Thinking You* knows is best.

1. Make a list of fun activities you can do when you feel bored, or when you want to eat but aren't really hungry.

2. Make a list of things you can do or people you can talk to when you are feeling sad, upset, or nervous and want to eat.

Chapter 6
Train Yip to Use
the Stomach Stop Sign

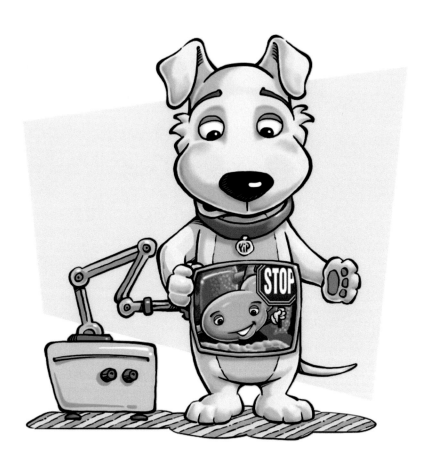

Help Yip learn to use his stomach as a STOP EATING sign.

Yip is used to eating as much food as he can find, or as much food as he wants. When food tastes good, it may be hard for Yip to notice as soon as his stomach feels JUST FULL. Remind Yip, "You can have more tasty food again later, when it is the right time to eat." Tell Yip "Good job!" *every* time he stops as soon as he is JUST FULL.

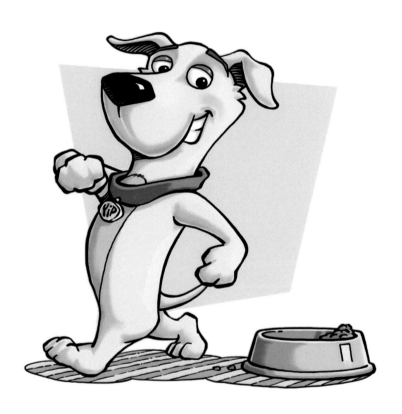

Help Yip walk away as soon as his stomach feels JUST FULL.

It may be hard for Yip to stop eating when there is still food in front of him. Yip may need to walk away from the food and find something else fun to do. Tell Yip "Good job!" *every* time he decides to stop eating as soon as his stomach is JUST FULL and chooses to read a book, watch a show, or play with a friend instead.

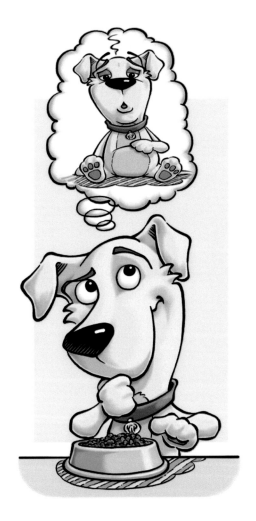

Help Yip remember his stomach doesn't feel so good when he eats a lot of sugar or gets STUFFED.

Puppies don't think about what happened yesterday. The *Thinking You* can help Yip be happy eating well by reminding him that eating a lot doesn't always feel good later. Tell Yip "Good job!" ***every*** time he remembers this lesson: Food tastes good, but getting STUFFED is NOT WORTH IT.

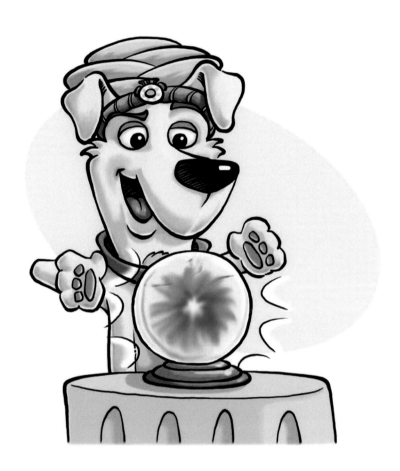

Help Yip think about the future.

Puppies don't think about how they will feel in a few minutes, how they will feel tomorrow, or how they will feel in a few weeks. The *Thinking You* can help Yip be happy eating well by reminding Yip that a healthier body feels so much better. Tell Yip "Good job!" ***every*** time he remembers this lesson: There are lots of fun things to do besides eating. If I stop eating when I am JUST FULL, I will feel better in my body.

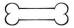

1. Remember a time when you ate so much that you didn't feel good. Draw a picture or write a story about the situation to help you remember it doesn't always feel good to eat a large amount.

2. Remember a time when you walked away or said "No, thank you" when you had already had enough treats. Draw a picture or write a story about how hard it is to say "NO" to tasty food and how good you feel when you don't eat too much.

Chapter 7
The Well-Trained Yip

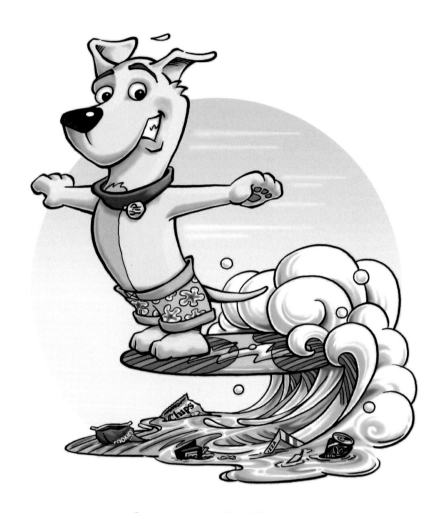

Yip lives in a FUN FOOD WORLD full of tasty treats.

Help Yip practice "surfing" when he sees a lot of tasty food and wants to eat. When you surf, you stay on top of the wave so you don't fall down into the water. You can learn to "ride out" an urge to eat tasty foods when you see them. Think of the urge to eat like a wave. The urge will go away in a few minutes if you JUST WAIT, or if you DISTRACT yourself by thinking about something else really interesting or fun.

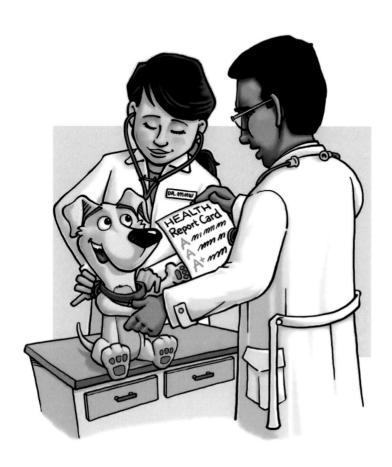

Congratulations! Your Inner Pup is now well trained.

What are the lessons Yip remembers to help him eat well and feel his best?

- Lesson One: "I know lots of ways to have fun and to feel better. I don't need to eat every time I want to eat."
- Lesson Two: "My body feels best when I stop at JUST FULL. My stomach doesn't feel so good when I have a lot of sugar or get STUFFED."
- Lesson Three: "When I want to keep eating more, I remember I can have more tasty food later when it is the right time to eat"

A well-trained Yip stops and thinks before eating. Most of the time he makes healthy choices.

What are Yip's new, healthy eating habits?

- Yip eats regular nutritious meals and snacks so he doesn't get too HUNGRY.
- Yip likes many nutritious foods. He doesn't choose drinks with sugar.
- Yip knows how to walk away from food when he is JUST FULL.
- Yip enjoys treats, but he doesn't beg for treats every day.
- Yip doesn't choose treats when he is very HUNGRY.
- Yip is happy having small treats.
- Yip uses the Hunger Meter to decide when it is the right time to eat and when it is best to do something else. He doesn't eat every time he wants to eat.
- Yip uses the Worth-It Scale to make healthier choices that taste good.
- Yip uses the Stomach Stop Sign to stop eating before he get STUFFED even when he wants to eat more.

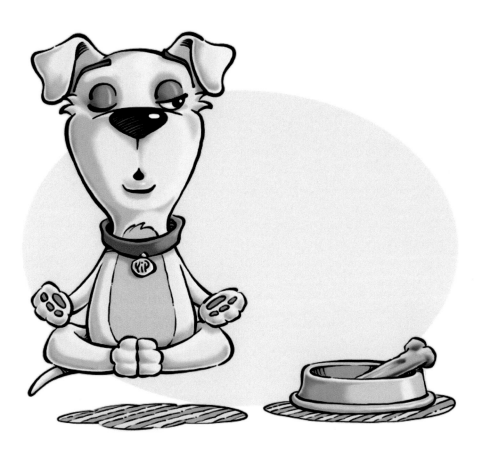

A well-trained Yip keeps practicing so he won't forget his new habits.

The *Thinking You* is still in charge of Yip, but you and Yip are now working together to be happy and stay healthy. Yip still likes to eat, and he likes treats. Sometimes he forgets his lessons and eats more than is healthy, but he remembers the next time. He tries hard to do what the *Thinking You* knows is best. The *Thinking You* has to be patient. Keep telling Yip "Good job!" *every* time he listens to his stomach and finds fun things to do besides eating.

Remember the story of the Tortoise and the Hare? Yip is like the tortoise. Yip keeps practicing every day. He doesn't stop to rest like the Hare. So, Yip will win the race to be happy and stay healthy.

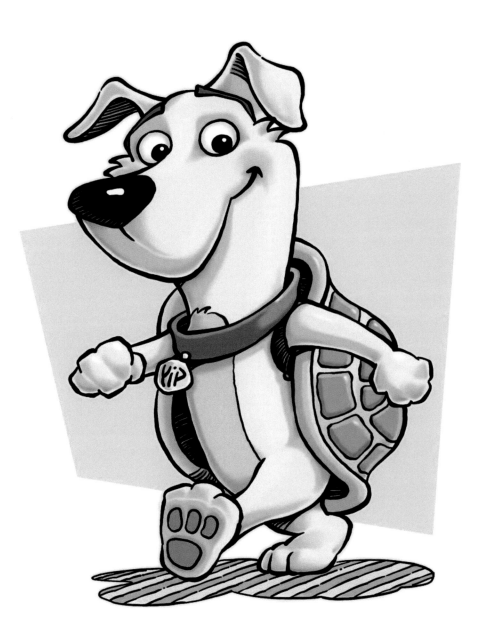

1.Practice JUST WAITING when it is not the right time to eat, or when you have already had a treat but you want more. Notice that it feels a little uncomfortable to JUST WAIT, but you can do it. It gets easier to JUST WAIT after you practice this skill a lot.

2.Draw a picture of your well-trained Yip and give him a gold star, or draw a gold star on this book when your Yip has learned to use the three tools (the *Hunger Meter*, the *Worth-It Scale*, and the *Stomach Stop Sign*). Put another gold star on your picture (or in the book) every week you keep training Yip. Remember, Yip has to keep using these tools every day to feel good and stay healthy. Remember to tell yourself "Good job!" *every* time you and Yip work together to make healthier choices.

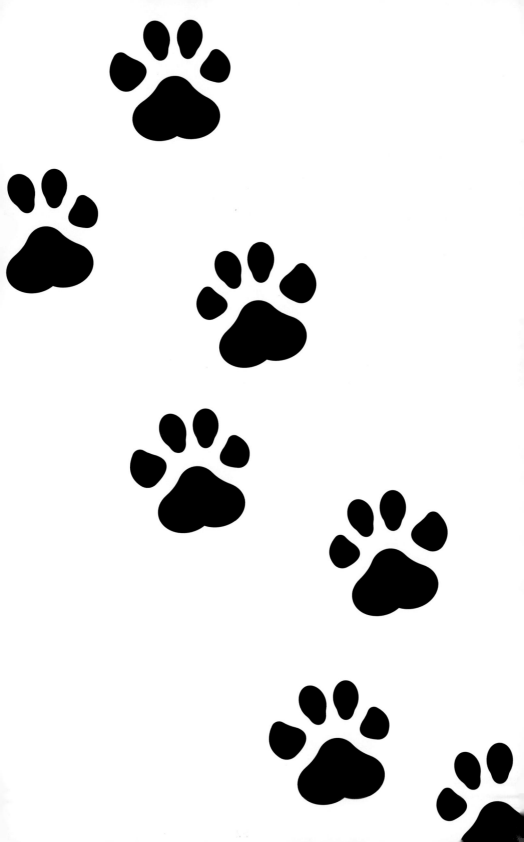

Glossary

Eating well: When you make choices about what and how much to eat that balance the pleasure you get from food with consideration of your health and well-being.

FUN FOOD WORLD: An environment in which tasty, cheap, high-calorie food is easily available and in which cultural norms support using food as a reward and as a central part of socializing and celebrations.

Grazing: A pattern of eating small to moderate amounts over an extended period of time, which can be problematic if you choose primarily treats instead of more nutritious foods, or if you end up having more calories over the whole day than you would have if you had just eaten regular nutritious meals and a few snacks.

Healthy choices/Healthy eating habits: When you eat nutritious foods most of the time and you also eat only moderate amounts, which allows you to maintain, or achieve, a medically healthy body.

HUNGRY versus want to eat: In this book, "HUNGRY" means you feel hungry in your stomach (this usually happens when you haven't eaten in a few hours; however, if you eat a very sugary treat without enough nutritious food, you may feel hungry sooner). In this book, "*want to eat*" means you aren't hungry in your stomach but you *want* some taste in your mouth (can also be described as *mouth hunger* or a *craving*).

JUST FULL: Refers to the very early signs of stomach distension. It is best to stop eating at this early sign because it takes a little while for your brain to process the signals from your stomach. When you stop at JUST FULL, you will feel comfortably full in fifteen minutes, whereas if you don't stop eating until you feel very definitely full, you are likely to feel a bit uncomfortably full in fifteen minutes.

JUST WAIT: A way to cope with urges to eat when you are not hungry; you can choose to tolerate the discomfort as an alternative to the strategy of deliberating distracting yourself with fun activities or thinking about something else besides food. As you practice JUST WAIT, you'll notice that urges to eat are naturally replaced by other thoughts coming into your mind. That is, unless you keep refocusing on thoughts about what you *want* to eat and remain upset that you can't have what you *want* to eat. Imagine an urge being like a snowflake landing on your hand; it will melt on its own if you leave it alone. Other snowflakes may replace it, but they, too, will melt on their own. You can squash the snowflake to make it go away, but it isn't necessary.

Let your stomach be your guide: When you make decisions based on your stomach sensations, not just on what your brain says you want to eat or what your mouth says will taste good.

Listening to your stomach: Paying attention to hunger and fullness sensations in your stomach; noticing the early signs that you are getting hungry, and choosing to have a meal or snack so you don't get so hungry you make less healthy choices; noticing the first signs of stomach distention and choosing to stop at JUST FULL.

NOT WORTH IT: When you notice that you regret what or how much you ate, but you notice this only *after* you have eaten it. The regret is typically that the food didn't actually taste that good (or at least not as good as you expected), or that you weren't paying attention and ate more than now feels comfortable (also called *mindless eating*).

Nutritious food: Meals or snacks that include a substantial amount of protein, complex carbohydrates/fiber, "good" fats, vitamins, or minerals rather than "empty calorie" foods that provide calories primarily from sugars, refined carbohydrates, and less healthy fats (e.g., junk food).

Riding out an urge: When you know you *want* to eat but decide not to, because it is not the right time to eat. You JUST WAIT. As you practice riding out urges, you notice that desires to eat may initially seem to get stronger, but like a wave, the urge will diminish over time. The idea is you don't have to satisfy every urge to eat that you experience.

Right time to eat: Regularly scheduled meals or snacks are the best times to eat. Eating at fairly consistent times over the day, even if you are not that hungry. Regular meals *prevent* getting so HUNGRY you have a hard time carefully considering healthier choices and stopping at JUST FULL.

Too HUNGRY: When you feel so hungry, you don't stop to think about what would be Worth It before you eat. You may eat whatever food is easiest to get, eat very fast, or eat more than you would if you had not been so hungry.

Trainer: A person with a certain expertise who takes responsibility for educating, preparing, and guiding another person (or animal) to develop certain skills, typically using hands-on, experiential methods.

Treats: Foods that you really like, so you are likely to eat larger amounts than is healthy for your body. Often—but not always—treats are highly processed foods lower in nutritional value (i.e., so-called "junk food").

WORTH IT: When you enjoyed what you ate and don't feel deprived, and you still feel good in your body after you have finished eating. WORTH IT generally means you were hungry so you needed to eat, or you really *wanted* a treat and were able to keep it to a small amount, so you felt good about your choice.

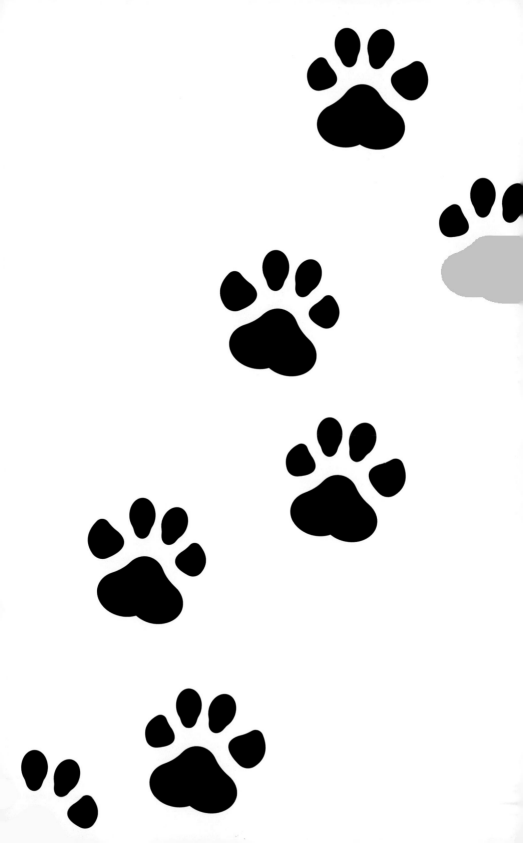

To my husband, Ed, who gave me the confidence to introduce Yip to children and their families everywhere, and to my grandchildren, Lily, Zoey, and Sawyer, who inspire me every day to enter their magical worlds and think like a child again.

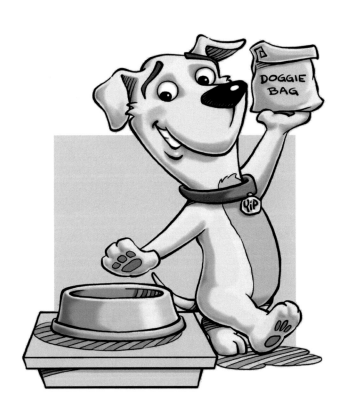

About the Author

Linda W. Craighead, PhD, is a professor of psychology at Emory University in Atlanta and director of the graduate training program in clinical psychology. Dr. Craighead received her BA from Vanderbilt University and her PhD in psychology from the Pennsylvania State University. She has been on the faculty at the Pennsylvania State University, the University of North Carolina at Chapel Hill, and the University of Colorado at Boulder. Dr. Craighead has published extensively in the area of eating disorders and weight concerns, and practices as a licensed clinical psychologist. She developed and evaluated an intervention described in *The Appetite Awareness Workbook* (New Harbinger, 2006) to help adults overcome binge eating, overeating, and preoccupation with food. Appetite awareness training (AAT) incorporates aspects of mindful eating into the well-established strategies of cognitive behavioral intervention for eating and weight problems. Dr. Craighead gives workshops, nationally and internationally, providing training in the application of appetite awareness and the use of mobile technology (apps) to a range of problems related to eating and weight.

Other Books by
Linda W. Craighead, PhD

The Appetite Awareness Workbook: How to Listen to Your Body and Overcome Binge Eating, Overeating, and Obsession with Food

Psychopathology: History, Diagnosis, and Empirical Foundations (3rd Edition)

Edited with David J. Miklowitz and W. Edward Craighead

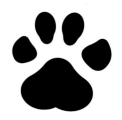

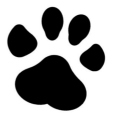

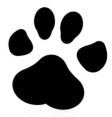